Made in the USA
Las Vegas, NV
02 May 2021

22366103R00057